Interface between Research and Practice

some working models

Barbara Vaughan
Mary Edwards

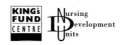

Published by the King's Fund Centre
126 Albert Street
London
NW1 7NF
Tel: 0171-267 6111

ISBN 1 85717 084 9

A CIP catalogue record for this book is available from the British Library

Distributed by:
Bournemouth English Book Centre (BEBC)
PO Box 1496
Parkstone
Poole
Dorset
BH12 3YD

The King's Fund Centre is a health services development agency which promotes improvements in health and social care. We do this by working with people in health services, in social services, in voluntary agencies, and with the users of their services. We encourage people to try out new ideas, provide financial or practical support to new developments, and enable experiences to be shared through workshops, conferences and publications. Our aim is to ensure that good developments in health and social care are widely taken up.

Contents

Foreword

At a time of unprecedented debate about the best way to organise and deliver health services, the need to strengthen the knowledge base of health care is one of the few topics on which there is consensus. The growing interest in methods of evaluating health care technologies and the processes of care has been matched by a new commitment to strengthen the research base, notably through the NHS Research and Development programme. The creation of new knowledge about clinical effectiveness and the synthesis and dissemination of existing knowledge are essential preconditions for improving the quality and appropriateness of health care, but they are not sufficient in themselves. If patients are to benefit from all this effort, equal attention will have to be paid to the implementation of evidence-based practice. This, coupled with the identification of research questions arising from the critical appraisal of everyday practice, sets a demanding agenda for practitioners.

This publication brings together a number of different approaches to the promotion of evidence-based practice arising from the practical experience of the King's Fund-supported Nursing Development Units. In describing the way in which the units have brought about changes in practice, ranging from attempts to stimulate an evidence-based culture, through practical implementation of research findings, to carrying out more formal research studies, the report highlights the achievements as well the difficulties faced by those trying to narrow down the gap between research and practice.

Changing clinical practice is never easy. It requires a willingness to challenge received wisdom and to rethink traditional ways of working. Success depends on effective leadership and powers of persuasion, as well as a sound grasp of the research evidence. In sharing these experience with a wider audience we hope to support those engaged in this task and help them to build on the work of the 30 NDUs. The approaches documented here provide ample evidence that change is possible. They demonstrate that practitioners, managers and researchers can work together to develop local strategies for change. It is beholden on all of us to ensure that the services which patients are offered are built on a sound knowledge base.

Angela Coulter, Director, King's Fund Centre

Preface

Ensuring that clinical care is based on sound knowledge is high on everyone's agenda within the current health service, and there are many local and national initiatives which have been established to address this need. While considerable attention has been paid to the dissemination of information, fewer initiatives have focused on how this information can be assimilated into day-to-day practice or indeed how practice itself can inform future research agendas.

This report has arisen from the experience of nurses and reserchers working in Nursing, Midwifery and Health Visiting Development Units (NDUs) throughout the UK (see the Appendix for a list of participants) who have explored ways of bringing research and practice together. It offers an overview of different approaches relating to the research–practice interface, ranging from research utilisation to development activities which may lead to the formulation of research questions and more formal research activity.

This work has been prepared for those who have an interest and responsibility to ensure that patient/client care is knowledge-based and a desire to extend their insight into the way in which nursing practice has an impact on the quality of care. It is not intended to be prescriptive in any way: the approaches explored are not mutually exclusive. Indeed, great emphasis has been placed throughout the report on the need to identify local aims and contextual constraints before deciding on a local strategy. The main purpose of this work is to stimulate debate, raise questions and identify points for consideration to help colleagues with similar aspirations.

Barbara Vaughan
Director
Nursing Developments Programme
King's Fund Centre

Mary Edwards
Clinical Effectiveness Manager
NHS Executive
South and West Regional Office

Acknowledgements

The King's Fund would like to acknowledge the NDU staff who have provided the ideas and experiences which are presented in this work. In particular, thanks are due to workshop participants (identified in the Appendix) whose help has been invaluable in clarifying the ideas presented here and commenting on draft copies of the publication.

One of the imperatives behind the Nursing, Midwifery and Health Visiting Development Units (NDUs) programme has been to enhance the quality of care offered to patients and clients through the use of knowledge-based practice. Alongside this, the NDUs also have a responsibility to evaluate the efficacy of their work. In line with this demand, several different models have emerged where an interface between research and practice occurs. This paper outlines the variety of approaches which have been taken to meet this end, highlighting the advantages and difficulties which the units have experienced, and raising issues for consideration when planning further local action. A discussion is included about the need to clarify expectations and desired outcomes when considering which approach to take.

National and local initiatives

At a national level, the drive to increase the use of research in practice is high.[1] This has been supported by initiatives such as the establishment of the Cochrane Collaboration,[2] which undertakes meta-analysis of randomised controlled trials (RCTs) on specific topics to make an overview more readily available to practitioners; and the York Centre for Review and Dissemination,[3] which has a similar remit but reviews a wider range of research; the drive for the use of audit in clinical practice;[4] and the establishment of national targets in relation to research implementation.[5]

However, if maximum benefit is to be gained from these activities, it is also necessary to develop implementation strategies which bring together research and practice. The models described in this publication are a demonstration of local initiatives which have been taken at the practice level to bring about changes in actual service delivery. The variety of approaches described reflects the variations in the units themselves; while they all share the common aim of improving patient care, the steps taken to achieve this vary according to local need and circumstances.

Clarifying the rationale

A further issue which has become apparent through work with the NDUs is the need to be clear about the rationale behind research-related activities. If this is not made explicit, then confusion can occur in terms of both expectation and action.

Three broad areas of activity can be identified which all have an important function but require different strategies. They are:

- research-based practice
- scientific research
- data to guide policy.

Research-based practice

The demand for a practice–research interface comes from the need to account for practice and ensure that the knowledge base on which clinical decisions are made is sound. The skills required here relate both to interpretation and use of research findings and to management of change. Thus the main purpose behind this approach is:

> *to ensure that practice is knowledge-based through the introduction and evaluation of research-based practice; to develop research and evaluation skills among clinical staff; and to create an ethos of enquiry.*

The work of both the early and the current NDUs suggests that the development of evaluative skills in the nursing team can have a direct impact on patient care through the manner in which it enhances application of research findings.[6] Charging members of the clinical team with the responsibility to explore the literature on a specific clinical topic (e.g. wound care, tissue viability, reminiscence, or immunisation) and thus developing them into a local source of knowledge for colleagues is a very effective way of enhancing local expertise. It also serves to heighten awareness of the need to underpin practice with knowledge.

Within this context, many units carry out small-scale 'research studies', more accurately called 'evaluation', to assess the efficacy of research-based practice using either care protocols or standards as a means of disseminating their work. As the *Report of the Task Force on the Strategy in Nursing, Midwifery and Health Visiting*[7] suggests:

> The term research is at times used in a rather loose and general way to describe a variety of activities and processes. We use the term 'research' to mean rigorous and systematic enquiry, conducted on a scale and using methods commensurate with the issue to be investigated and designed to lead to generalisable contributions to knowledge.

Care does have to be taken, however, that implementation and evaluation are carried out with good supervision as the processes involved are just as rigorous. There is in fact a risk of becoming too prescriptive or of overloading the clinical areas with investigative studies.

Scientific research

Any profession which offers a service to others needs to develop the knowledge base which forms the foundation of judgement and decision making. Thus in nursing, one vital rationale for research and evaluation generated from practice is the need to add to the body of scientific knowledge which underpins nursing, and this requires a rigorous scientific approach.

Studies of this kind are essential to the future of nursing and it is of critical importance that opportunities are found which allow for their development. However, by its very nature, this work is lengthy and even though interim reports can be produced, findings are frequently not available for several years. There can be a tension between the time needed to undertake research of this nature and the shorter time available for decision makers to plan and bring about change, and these varying demands can lead to considerable strain for those involved. There are also cost implications related to the time span as well as a need to ensure that the requisite skills are available to guarantee academic credibility.

Data to guide policy

As changes are occurring so rapidly, there are times when information on which to base policy is required with some degree of urgency. Thus a further reason for carrying out evaluative work is to gather evaluative data to guide policy.

In this instance, it is possible to identify information which can be gathered over a shorter time span and which can be of either a quantitative or a qualitative nature. Surveys can be carried out and data collated relatively quickly about such items as variations in length of stay, throughput, contact times and staff attendance. Similarly, clinical data can be gathered about items such as skin integrity, pain severity or incidence of disturbed behaviour.

Local needs

What are the local needs and expectations in relation to the research–practice interface? Is the main aim to increase the use of research in practice and evaluate its impact, or is there a broader remit to undertake new research? A continuum of needs can be identified which serve a number of different purposes. These can be classified as follows.

- **Research awareness** – where a *critical* enquiring approach to practice is taken and questions are raised about the rationale behind day-to-day practices.
- **Research use** – where steps are taken to bring about changes in practice which are founded on sound evidence based on research and applied critically in context.
- **Evaluation** – where the impact of changes in practice is systematically evaluated against predefined goals. This may then be followed by monitoring through a quality-improvement programme or audit.
- **Development work** – where the feasibility of new approaches to practice is explored. These may become the subject of more rigorous research at a later date.
- **Research activity** – where a clear research question has been identified and becomes the subject of formal enquiry.

Being clear about expectations helps to establish which strategies should be taken; what skills are required; what outcomes can be expected; and in what time frame they can be achieved.

In some models, the introduction of research-based practice and its evaluation are the aim rather than undertaking formal research. This approach can lead to the development of role models of good practice and care protocols which are sensitive to local circumstances, and can be used by others within the host organisation. The units which work in this way are fundamentally *development units*, concerned with the use of knowledge in practice and evaluation of the changes. The services that they offer are of great value at a local level in improving the quality of patient care. Much can also be learned from the processes which they have used to achieve these ends, and sharing these experiences through publications and conference presentations can act as a strong motivator to encourage less experienced units to 'try it for themselves'.

In other models, there is a move to more analytical work on the development of nursing with a greater emphasis on the research end of the continuum. Here, new ideas may be tried and tested or clarification of some aspects of nursing sought. The outcome of this work is of great value, not only in improving services but also in adding to our understanding of the way in which nurses can contribute to service delivery. Although work of this nature takes time before formal outcomes are available to the wider audience, the long-term gains are high and may result in new methods and strategies emerging. (See Fig.1.)

RESEARCH–PRACTICE CONTINUUM

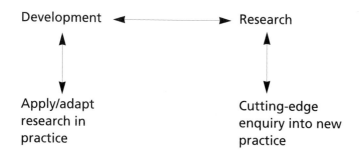

Fig.1

Linking research, learning and audit to improve clinical effectiveness

The ultimate aim of changing the behaviour of practitioners is to improve patient care through increasing their clinical effectiveness. This will need not only sound research findings but also various strategies to encourage practitioners to *implement* that research evidence. Learning and clinical audit can help achieve this end.

Learning

Learning is taken here as the process through which new knowledge is internalised by an individual. This may take place through formal education (e.g courses and workshops on specific topics) or it may happen in a more informal way in the workplace as has been the case in many of the NDUs. There is a growing recognition of the need to encourage and support the continuing professional development of health professionals, reflected in the UKCC's requirements[8] and some of the medical Royal Colleges' systems of cognate points, much of which can take place in the workplace rather than requiring costly courses that take staff away from work. Such a perspective is reflected in some of the models described below. There is also evidence that practitioners learn more effectively when this is associated with their real job tasks rather than theoretical activities in isolation.[9]

Clinical audit

Clinical audit, which monitors standards of practice, can also be seen as part of this cycle. Indeed, this is one of its principal characteristics according to the Department of Health.[10] It can be linked to portfolio learning where individuals indicate their particular development needs and develop plans to meet those educational objectives. This again would fit with the concept of PREPP[11] and other similar mechanisms for professional updating. There is great potential for learning to take place at all stages of the audit cycle and this should be emphasised as teams develop their audit programmes.

Therefore if the three concepts – research, learning and audit – are linked in a co-ordinated fashion, the outcome should be more effective clinical practice and service provision. This results in a situation where the research process produces sound evidence, which is translated into user-friendly information (e.g. clinical guidelines), which is in turn introduced to practitioners through an educational process and monitored through the audit process (see Fig.2). Practice itself can inform the future research agenda ensuring its relevance to patient care.

Determine the nature of best practice

Inform professionals/ clinical team of development and promote uptake into clinical practice

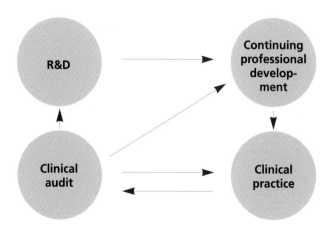

Assessment of effectiveness of implementation and patient benefit

Implementation of learned best practice, perhaps through guidelines

Fig.2

Thus clinical audit can be used to demonstrate that the individual and team are achieving the research-based standards; to enhance the learning process; and to identify areas for development which may become the focus of future research activity.

Conclusion

The models described here are not mutually exclusive and in some units advantage has been taken of more than one approach to ensure that different aspects of enquiry are meet. What is common to all the approaches is an ethos of enquiry which, once established, is self-perpetuating, leading to a shift from rule-bound practice to a service which is flexible, creative, thoughtful and patient-centred. Furthermore, if public accountability for practice is a requirement of any service provider, then ways of enhancing the knowledge base of practice become both an ethical and an organisational imperative.

Summary of principles

1 Before identifying strategies to develop the research–practice interface, it is essential that the purpose behind such activities is clarified with note taken of the current stage of development within both the team and the organisation.

2 As different skills are required in different roles, there is a need to clarify the specific expertise required in new roles.

3 Similarly, it is important to clarify the boundaries of responsibility and authority, with lines of accountability and working relationships agreed by all involved.

4 Ways of providing academic supervision need to be sought for those with responsibility for research and/or evaluation in order to ensure both academic credibility and personal support.

5 Role overload can be a real problem requiring negotiation of responsibilities and the provision of appropriate support (e.g. administrative support and resourced time).

6 If change is to be truly effective, it is essential to involve all the clinical team in order that they can gain ownership of the initiatives.

7 Ethical consideration must be given not only to the research process but to the expectations of those involved and to the consequences of *not* investing in developing the research–practice interface.

8 There is a need to clarify the relationship between research, evaluation, audit and development and the manner in which they interrelate.

9 When planning local strategies, it is important to take contextual issues into consideration, recognising that none of the approaches described here is mutually exclusive and novel combinations to meet local need may be developed.

10 The value of practice development and research utilisation is as high as more formal research enquiry and as demanding to achieve. Thus equal attention needs to be paid to resourcing and supporting each end of the continuum of initiatives.

In order to gain an accurate
description of the models considered
below we sought help from a group
of practitioners and researchers who
are actively involved in the different
approaches (see the Appendix). Both
the advantages and difficulties where
explored through group work
and the quotes used arise directly
from this work. In this way, we hope
to have captured an honest picture
of what can be achieved through
a variety of different mechanisms,
as well as exploring realistic
expectations. In each section, the issue
of resources has been raised in order
that it can be weighed against
expected outcomes.

Model I
Internal evaluation within the NDU team

This could be described as the 'getting going' approach where, under the leadership and guidance of the clinical leader, the team identify areas of practice which will be the focus of development. The work is largely internal and is closely linked with staff development and implementation of previously validated work. It may be seen as a catalyst for change.

Audit tools are frequently used within this context as a means of identifying both strengths and weaknesses in current practice. For example, an audit of documents may lead to recognition that record-keeping is inadequate and that the documents themselves are not flexible enough to reflect individual client need. Similarly, quality assessment tools such as QUALPACS[12] may be used diagnostically to this end.

Alternatively, individual performance review may be employed to identify personal interests which are of relevance to the whole unit.[13] In the same way, clinical supervision may highlight a learning need which can be met through developing the knowledge and skills of practitioners.[14] Thus the model is essentially practitioner/client-led, drawing on the experiences and needs of the local situation and offering opportunity for personal development.

Linked to identification of developmental needs is an action plan which may include such activities as a literature search, development of a standard or protocol, preparation of a resource file or development of a local 'expert'. In the early days, the clinical leader may undertake some of this work as a role-model but as skills develop so the responsibility can be devolved.

Time may be freed in a number of different ways. In one instance, a part-time team member has been employed to give time out for colleagues to undertake such work. Alternatively, the team have managed their off-duty to allow specified time to be allotted to this work within their establishment, although this is becoming increasingly difficult.

Essentially, this approach provides a systematic ongoing process which involves the whole team and supports the introduction of research-based practice as well as enhancing personal development.

The model concentrates strongly on use of research and evaluation of its impact on practice, but as the participants said, '*You have to check that the change is really appropriate – you cannot ignore it – you need to demonstrate that it works.*'

Strengths of the model

For the clinical team

This is a very pragmatic approach which involves the whole team and generates a feeling of ownership and self-worth. It can have a very positive impact on staff morale and team building since there is opportunity for meeting both unit and personal aims. As participants said, '*We need to recognise the value of the work we do – for credibility*', and this is one way of achieving that end.

Because the ideas are generated internally, the relevance and therefore the value of the work can be easily recognised. '*The team have total control of it – if you are part of the team you actually own the work.*' While there is an acknowledgement that this approach is nearer to implementation than research, it is a powerful way of developing practice and gaining insight into the research process.

For the participants

People who have been involved in this approach speak of the increased job satisfaction. They see it as a way of developing their critical thinking ability as well as increasing their understanding of the research process. They speak of a '*process of internalisation ... where involvement in internal evaluation is a preparation for the future.*'

There is also a high value placed on the formal, legitimate opportunity to take time out to explore a particular issue which the team recognise as being important to their practice. '*As the practitioner is so close to the client, the issues covered arise directly out of practice. What nurses at ground level need is to get really confident.*'

This approach is also seen as a way of getting minority groups who may resist change involved. There is a view that it offers the opportunity of '*getting closer to those groups and making sure that their perceptions are really represented'*, since it is internal and therefore less threatening.

For clinical care

Because of the continuing clinical work, there is an opportunity to gain insight into the true impact of any changes for patients, and to involve the team in some of the processes. Assumptions can be challenged which have been taken for granted. There is also the chance to deal with small issues which can be lost in larger research work, such as environmental factors which cause discomfort to patients.

Essentially, participants strongly believe (evidenced by their local evaluation) that internal evaluation can have an impact on the quality of patient care and, as they say, *'if it has an impact on patient care, it makes it all worthwhile.'*

Difficulties with the model

For the clinical team

For the clinical team the greatest difficulty with this model is that the evaluation gets 'squeezed out' by clinical priorities and it is more difficult to get dedicated time. As they say, *'There is the added frustration of day-to-day work, added to which it can be difficult to remain objective.'* As there is no direct line into a validating body, it can be difficult to obtain recognition for the work undertaken although, with the advent of PREPP[15] and processes for accreditation of prior learning, there are now ways in which this can be done.

For the researcher/evaluator

In this instance, the researcher/evaluators are part of the clinical team, so many of the difficulties are shared. However, an added concern is the need for expertise in research methods which is not always readily available. As internal evaluation is seen as a means of assuring the validity of actions, it is critical that the work can stand the test of scrutiny. Thus there is a need to be sure of the process used. One way of overcoming this is to use previously validated methods, that is to *replicate* work at a local level. In this way, previous work can be built on and both the reliability and validity of the approach taken become stronger.

For clinical care

The difficulties in relation to clinical care are primarily concerned with time, since it can be difficult to prioritise. There is also some risk that as expertise develops in one practitioner it is not shared with others, but this can be overcome with well-planned mechanisms for using team members as local consultants.

Discussion

In this model, there is a real opportunity to highlight the value of research from a practitioner's perspective. It makes visible the impact of changes in practice since '*you need to analyse whether that change has really had any effect.*' As those involved say, '*The fact that someone comes in from outside – you are not necessarily going to take them by the hand and say "I'm going to do this". This way it is more flexible and relevant – the fact that we are involved increases the relevance and gives you more energy.*'

The need to share experiences of research use and evaluation was also highlighted. '*The more areas in which a subject is explored, the more credibility it has. If it is published then other people start to think "I could do that", which makes practice development much more realistic.*'

A further opportunity which this model offers is for practitioners to gain insight into the world of research and learn to recognise the value of knowledge-based practice. A ripple effect can occur where, once one area of practice has been challenged, others will also be questioned.

This is probably the least threatening model of all, since it is practice-driven and arises from the work of the whole team. In some instances, it has been difficult to 'get everyone on board' with an attitude that the work is for others, when all the classic signs of resistance to change are seen. However, through involvement, holding people to account and positive feedback, such a situation can usually be overcome.

It also has to be borne in mind that this is not the approach to take when major research work is required and in some cases there have been unrealistic expectations of what can be achieved by a team who have neither the resources nor the skills to undertake new research nor to take full responsibility for dissemination throughout the rest of the organisation. Thus if the work is to have maximum impact, links with managers and teachers to meet these ends are needed.

Resources

This model is less demanding on resources than some of the others, but great care has to be taken to ensure that the time needed is seen as 'legitimate' and hence costed. It is also important that the relevant skills are available to ensure that the evaluation is reliable.

Transferability

While the model here has been described from a nursing perspective, it can also be very effective when an issue is explored from a multiprofessional stance which is, in reality, often the case. In this way, it can do much to enhance interdisciplinary relationships and help all members of the team to learn about individual contributions.

As those involved say, '*We need to be aware of research principles when we are changing practice, and internal evaluation leads to this. We need to demonstrate that it is not just a good idea, plucked from the sky – that the work we do is valid.*'

Model 2
The researcher as part of the NDU team

In this model, a researcher, who may or may not be a nurse, works directly within the unit as part of the team. Employment is within the Trust or health authority with accountability to the clinical leader/manager. Responsibilities are primarily to undertake rigorous research and/or evaluative work on behalf of the unit. There is, however, a secondary responsibility to help develop research expertise in other members of the NDU team.

The context

According to those involved in this approach, it has greatest value '*in units where some work has already been done ... to establish a good base line.*' They all suggest that their work has evolved over a period of time and in some cases, as greater insight has been gained into the unit's needs and expectations, '*the goalposts have moved*'. This emphasises the need for a clinical team with some experience in order that they can be clear from the outset about the nature of the work and hence the skills required to fulfil it. As one of them said, '*We didn't really know what we were taking on – employing someone (in the early stages) but now it is a huge relief because of the work pressure to have someone working alongside us.*'

Whether or not the researcher should be a nurse is open to debate; there are advantages and disadvantages on both sides, and neither is *intrinsically* preferable. As one nurse said, '*I am not sure that a non-nurse would not be more effective – as I get drawn into the clinical side of things.*' Alternatively, as a nurse, there has been the opportunity to help formulate the research questions and the direction of the project with inside knowledge of what needs to be achieved. Indeed, everyone involved stressed how important it was to get both the timing and the question right, taking into account external changes within the health service and new directions in the provision of services.

For the non-nurses, there are also clear advantages. As one said, '*I ask questions which possibly wouldn't occur to nurses – which may even seem a little naive but which help the nurses to explain more clearly what they are doing.*' They can see the world of nursing as it is seen by others and can retain a greater degree of objectivity.

At the end of the day, the critical factor in deciding whether the researcher should be a nurse is linked to the nature of the question being asked or the type of research required. The opportunity to formulate the research question is not dependent on the researcher's background, but on their relationship with the nursing team, the degree of autonomy the researcher has within the team and the team's autonomy within the clinical environment.

Strengths of the model

For the clinical team

'*To begin with, we saw the role as an outsider, but now we see you as one of us.*' This seems to say it all, as over a period of time the relevance of the research skills brought to the unit becomes apparent. Expertise is available directly to the staff and, as the researcher is part of the team, the work is integrated more readily. Communication between everyone involved is easier to maintain since the researcher is well known to the team. They speak of '*making research visible … demystifying it and providing bridges*' and see the researcher as '*a resource for others, only an office or telephone call away.*'

For the researcher

From the researcher's point of view much is gained from being part of a clinical team with direct insight into practice. Because of the close working relationship, they are in a strong position to ensure that their work remains grounded in reality, since they themselves are part of the context. There is opportunity for both planned and informal interaction which helps to paint a fuller picture. '*Short, off-the-cuff remarks over coffee and you can say "Ah – that is really important … I hadn't thought of that".*' As they see it, going hand in hand with the practitioners means that the two aspects are almost synonymous,

Model 2
The researcher as part
of the NDU team

and this helps to maintain a hold on the purpose of the work and protects the integrity of the research.

They add that the job is also fun, since it is very varied. Being part of the service and the decision making is seen as a major advantage with so many opportunities to learn from each other and contribute to the development work as well as the research.

A huge advantage is that the researcher gets to know the patients personally, '*as people, rather than numbers or letters on a computer screen; the work remains grounded in reality and this model ensures, to a large extent, that first and foremost the work is clinically, rather than academically, valuable.*'

For clinical care

As the relationship with both the clinical leader and the rest of the team develops so can the influence on practice. As one said, '*The impact of information on practice happens straightaway — it is so immediate. Having a member of the team with research expertise is very pervasive, affecting everything you do. It makes you think more carefully about everything you do.*' As they see it, there is also a better chance to get to know the patients and hence take their views and ideas into consideration when one is seen as part of the clinical team.

Difficulties with the model

For the clinical team

The greatest difficulty for the clinical team has occurred when the researcher has had to move on. The 'parting' with someone who has become integral to the unit brings with it problems. There can also be some concern from junior or new members of the team and care has to be taken that they do not see themselves as 'study objects'. Inevitably, there can also be a conflict in terms of priorities when the clinical demands outweigh the research ones. As they say, '*It is very easy to get caught up with the issues which are immediate*' and put to one side the research endeavour, losing sight of its real purpose and seeing it as '*nothing more than dull data collection.*'

For the researcher

For the researcher, the greatest risk has been in 'going native' and becoming so immersed in the work of the unit that objectivity can be lost. Strategies which can help reduce the risk include: having a separate office away from the ward where they can 'escape' and retain a balanced view, or seeking outside supervision.

There is also the difficulty of getting the right balance between the demands for quantitative data, especially from other members of the clinical team, and the need for qualitative approaches to nursing issues. There is a risk that they will be seen to be biased as they are part of the team, leading to an even greater need for rigour in the research design.

Isolation from research colleagues must also be guarded against as must the temptation to resist becoming a universal resource for the whole team. Thus academic supervision is an important consideration here in order to gain an objective view. Feelings of guilt can also exist in relation to the pressures on staff time and the need to contain the workload of the unit.

For clinical care

From a clinical perspective, the disadvantages are few although again care must be taken that the patients themselves are not 'over-researched.' To some extent the guilt of prioritising between care and research could be a risk but this is not great.

Discussion

This model offers a wide range of opportunities. It demystifies research at a clinical level, demonstrating what is achievable and meaningful in practice. Interestingly for the non-nurses not understanding some aspects of the work initially is seen as a very positive opportunity in that in clarifying what is happening you can *'reveal aspects of nursing which have been hidden for years and make them visible to people.'*

The partnership also means that the actual research question is informed by practice, ensuring its legitimacy and relevance. In turn,

Model 2
The researcher as part
of the NDU team

the impact on practice is high since there is a greater opportunity to see from the outset the applicability of the work.

The participants strongly emphasised the need for the researcher and the clinical team to share common values and beliefs, stressing the need for very careful selection. Choice at this stage is seen as crucial as well as the opportunity to clarify what is wanted from the project. As they said, '*If this stage is missed out you can be in big trouble*', since there may be a lack of understanding between those concerned.

Inevitably, there are also some threats to consider. Concern can arise over conflicts of interest, especially when some of the messages arising from the work are unexpected and not always easily accepted.[16] Nevertheless this can also be seen in a positive light as, from the researcher's angle, belonging to the team offers a greater chance to manage the way in which new insights are shared and strategies developed to bring about change.

Balancing the needs of the team with obligations to the organisation can also be difficult at times. From a medical perspective, '*science and hard research are the thing*' and persuading people of the value of qualitative work can be difficult. '*However once you get quality results, you are more likely to get resources but these have to be linked to the outcomes of the work*'.

What cannot be denied is that this role is '*incredibly hard work*'. Care has to be taken to retain a balance between personal needs (e.g. family life); personal aims, such as gaining an academic qualification; and the demands of the project work itself. Great support can also be gained through team membership with access which would not be available under other circumstances.

Resources

The obvious resource implication for this model is the salary for the researcher as well as some demand on other members of the team's time. However, this has to be weighed against the outcome, which gives rise to increase in both research utilisation and rigorous study.

Transferability

This approach is by no means limited to nursing and has already been well tried and tested in medical education through the research registrar post. Bringing researchers and practitioners together in this way can be used in either unidisciplinary or multidisciplinary work. Researchers in this model tend to carry out a fair amount of work with other departments in the unit, allowing the NDU to be a real resource to the organisation. This out-reach work provides a constant stimulus for the researcher; hard work but very rewarding.

There is one word of caution here. One of the strongest points the participants made was the importance of ensuring that there were shared values and beliefs, not only about patient care but also about the relevance of varying research methods. Since different occupational groups within the multidisciplinary team may well hold different views, there is a need for careful background work in establishing a programme which would encompass the varying contributions which can be made.

One final comment in relation to this model. It is seen as *a great opportunity to make nursing visible and valued.*

Model 3
Clinical fellows

This model offers a real opportunity for clinical nurses to become involved with research and development activity from a clinical base. Essentially, time is allocated for a team member to explore a clearly identified area of practice while retaining a reduced clinical input which can be achieved in a number of different ways. One approach has been to give team members a day a week out from their clinical responsibilities in six-monthly rotation to contribute to an ongoing project which was previously agreed by the team. Each person can identify and explore areas which are relevant to both the clinical sites concerned and individual interest. The work is co-ordinated by a facilitator to ensure continuity and guide the fellows. A high degree of involvement and ownership can be achieved in this way.

In another unit a full year's fellowship has been created, open to competition from the team. In this instance, it was the responsibility of the clinical fellow to identify which area of practice would be developed and explored.

In both cases, the people concerned stress the value of combining their clinical work with the development. As they see it, *'This is a clinical, not an academic fellowship, which brought the focus back to clinical work.'*

Strengths of the model

For the clinical team

The greatest advantage for the clinical team as a whole is the opportunity to take ownership of the work. They see the fellowships, which are relatively new to nursing, *'as a way of valuing nursing, of giving it recognition and of the recognition of clinical expertise'*. They also see it as a way of demonstrating how advanced clinical roles can be developed which contribute to the quality of the nursing service. As the work has progressed, there is a strong feeling among the team that they can demonstrate to others just what can be achieved, given the time and opportunity. In their words, '*It has sent a message right through our organisation that people can be recognised for their expert nursing skills.*'

In both the approaches, the fellows themselves have become a resource for the rest of their colleagues as their knowledge and expertise has grown in a specific practice area. It should be added that this is not contained within nursing and as one said, '*even medics have sought advice*'.

Maybe the strongest message is that since the team themselves generated the ideas, '*the system enabled ownership to come from the team ... since they had a vested interest in its success. For the rest of the clinical team, just seeing it done acts as a strong motivator which in turn impacts on the rest of their work.*' Thus an ethos of what *can* be done is created.

For the fellows

There is no doubt that for the clinical fellows themselves this has been a very positive experience which has impacted on both their professional and personal lives. It has provided an excellent chance for personal development with insight into and ownership of the value of research, but has also helped them to gain confidence in their own ability and to see ways in which they can contribute to practice development.

They emphasise the advantage of retaining their clinical responsibilities while undertaking this work. Since they were still part of the clinical team they could see where the strengths and weaknesses lay and thus concentrate their efforts. More importantly, the rest of the team could provide support for them personally, especially as they began to see the impact of the work and future opportunities. This peer support is further enhanced where there is more than one clinical fellow. Similarly, if the fellows work in a number of different clinical settings, there are opportunities to network across specialities. As they see it, '*nurses very quickly grasped the idea that this was something we could do for ourselves*', and while dangers of elitism could have arisen, in reality this was not the case.

For clinical care

As far as patients are concerned, there are several very specific outcomes. First, the focus of the work which the clinical fellows undertake leads to an increase in the use of knowledge-based practice either through the development and evaluation of a specific practice initiative or through the introduction of local 'experts'. There is also opportunity for them to contribute to the work in progress and have some influence on its direction and validation.

On a broader front, the introduction of the clinical fellows has had an impact on the ethos of the whole unit, leading to a spirit of enquiry and willingness to challenge practice. Questions are raised which could form the basis of a larger research study in the future. This opens up the chance to explore either new services or the impact of nursing interventions on patient outcomes, all of which help to raise the standards of care.

Difficulties with the model

For the clinical team

As the work can be seen as 'pioneering' at a clinical level, it brings with it some of the difficulties which are present in any change situation. For example, there may be some conflict arising between the demands of day-to-day practice for the team and the support that they are asked to give to the fellows. Similarly, as the work of the fellows emerges, there are implications for each team member to consider and in some instances a need to change practice at a personal level. Sometimes they have difficulty in seeing the long-term benefits of other people's work to become apparent.

Similar issues were raised in relation to nurse management where there were expectations that the impact of the work would be seen more quickly than is in fact the case.

For the clinical fellows

Even though the clinical fellows remain part of the clinical team, they can experience feelings of isolation as well as a degree of conflict between their dual responsibilities. They speak of the difficulties they have had in gaining recognition of their work and seeing their own progress. In the early days, the value of having the support of an external organisation (in this instance the King's Fund) in helping them to recognise their own achievements and ensure that these were also understood by senior managers was great.

There is a high pressure on the clinical fellows to be seen to be achieving, coupled with a fear of failure and of letting colleagues down. Since funding was used to back this work, they were acutely aware of the responsibilities which were not always immediately evident. As they say, '*It takes a while to see the difference.*' They also comment on the pressure on new people who will follow in their footsteps with an ever-increasing demand to achieve to a higher standard.

A final issue which needs to be raised in this section is the importance of ensuring that good supervision is available to the clinical fellows. Where a specific new approach to practice is being developed, clinical supervision may need to be external to the unit if expertise is not immediately available. In terms of the methodology used for both development and evaluation, it is critical that advice is readily at hand either through an internal facilitator or an external academic source.

For practice

The major difficulty from a clinical perspective is working within the reality of constraints arising from limited resources and a need to prioritise. As the degree of knowledge about 'what could be' increases, so the concern about what is possible also becomes apparent. Despite this, there is a strong counter-argument that it is only with knowledge that good decisions can be made when services have to be prioritised and there is strength through knowledge of being able to influence future service delivery patterns.

Discussion

A major opportunity which this model offers is to tap the energy and expertise of all the team members whatever their current roles may be. Since access is open to all, it is seen as a real way to take practice forward within the bounds of professional accountability, which is neither hierarchial nor constrained in any way by the boundaries of a course. At one end of the continuum, it provides a chance to increase the use of knowledge-based practice which may well act as the foundation for more formal research. Thus it sets the foundations for the next stage of enquiry. At the other end of the continuum, it creates the chance to seek out new services which can be developed and tested in a safe environment.

A further opportunity which they see is the freedom to define the development to match clinical needs without being influenced by any external 'hidden agendas'. While it would be foolhardy not to recognise the contextual changes within health care, it is also important to create windows of opportunity for exploring and developing innovative ideas, and this model gives just such a chance.

Interestingly, the threats were not seen in the model of clinical fellow itself but in the content of some of their work. For example, if research-based protocols were being developed against which clinical outcomes could be assessed in the long term, there would be obvious implications for changes in practice for the whole team. In some instances, the developments have brought to light limited practice and, in line with the audit–research–learning cycle, the need for learning opportunities to be made available is apparent. Turning this to a positive light, such knowledge can form the basis of an educational programme both within the unit and for the wider Trust teams.

Seeking ways in which the work of clinical fellows can contribute on a wider basis has become of major importance. Strategies which have been used include workshops were the expertise can be shared, use of some of the protocols developed in other units, links with training departments to contribute to their programme of work, publications and conference presentations.

Getting managers 'on board' and helping them to gain insights into the long-term value of such a scheme as this is undoubtedly important, with a need to differentiate between the general need for professional development and the specific advantages inherent in clinical fellowships of developing expertise. Nevertheless as the work becomes more visible, this becomes less problematic.

Resources

As is always the case, there are financial implications in introducing this model which relate both to 'time out' for the fellows and the provision of supervision. One way of meeting this end is to form a liaison with a local educational institution if the skills are not available within the team. There is, however, a strong feeling that given the opportunity to prove its worth it can be seen as good investment of money since the resource implications can be outweighed by the outcomes.

Transferability

It is not unusual to see examples from other disciplines of the combination of clinical and research responsibilities. These posts, however, have generally been confined to working within their own uniprofessional groups, but much would be gained by seeking a multiprofessional perspective. This would be advantageous to clinical team development and cost effectiveness.

A final word from one of the fellows, '*We need to convince people of its worth. Once they can see, they will have no doubt.*'

Model 4
Unified roles

This model is characterised by one person having overall responsibility for both clinical direction and research projects. There is no single role that depicts this 'unified' approach because each one is developed differently to reflect both local service organisation and individual skills. As incumbents say, *'We have had to find a new way of working which encompasses multiple responsibilities.'* There is the potential for this model to be seen as the early development of the 'advanced practice' model which will enable the further development of clinical career pathways.

The dual responsibility is most commonly invested in the clinical leader, who manages both the unit and the research which, in consequence, are well integrated and feed off one another. Another approach has been to develop a 'job share' where two team members have taken the shared responsibility for delivery of clinical care and leading a specific aspect of research or evaluation. In this way, they have the opportunity of retaining and developing their clinical expertise but also enhancing their skills of enquiry, *'which offers an excellent career opportunity and retains a foot in both camps'*. An action research model is popular in this approach which allows for flexibility in choice of methods and high involvement of the team. Again, this offers an excellent model for development and involvement.

The unified model is thus seen to integrate the roles of education, research, consultancy, practice, supervision and management; clinical practice, however, is seen as the focus. The role is that of the expert practitioner and leader who is testing out existing knowledge and theory in a practical setting. It was the approach taken in the first Nursing Development Unit in Burford and led to the early work related to the use of nursing beds.[17]

Strengths of the model

The strengths of the model include the ability to integrate clinical experience within the researcher role which should therefore mean that the resulting research is grounded in, and relevant to, clinical practice. This arises because the researcher can identify topics and issues which are pertinent to clinical practice, not just of interest, and also determine appropriate methodologies.

For the clinical team

As far as the clinical team is concerned, the advantages relate to '*keeping clinical experts as part of the team and having readily accessible research skills available*'. This is of benefit in terms of providing advice on research projects, as well as understanding the results of research and translating these into practice. The individual will also be well placed to lead education for the team on research methodology and applying research results to enhance the total knowledge and skills of the team. As team members suggest, '*This is a real added bonus for the team when we are looking for ways to improve clinical practice.*'

For the researcher/practitioner

As far as the actual researcher/practitioner is concerned, there is the benefit of being seen as a credible member of the clinical team, in touch with the realities of clinical practice. This can make their lives much easier in terms of co-operation and access when undertaking research. If this role is seen as the embryo of advanced practice, it will also enhance an individual's career pathway still within clinical practice. This clearly has the added bonus of increased job satisfaction and motivation and provides the opportunity to keep clinical experts within the clinical field. In their view, albeit challenging, the role offers '*the chance to stay close to patients while developing expertise in other aspects of nursing work which are essential for the future.*'

For clinical care

The greatest advantage for patients in using this model is that they have continuing access to experienced practitioners who may otherwise be lured away into the world of research. The continuing presence of skilled researchers/practitioners not only has an influence on other members of the team but also ensures that research questions arise from a sound understanding of the reality of practice, opening up the opportunity for inductively generated ideas.

Difficulties with the model

For the clinical team

Creating a joint role such as this can create boundary issues for the individual in the team, particularly where there is already confusion between team members about role boundaries. These types of post are still quite new and the concept may be challenged by other professionals in the team. Both of these issues, dissonance and role boundary, require the incumbents to have a clear view about their roles and to make that view explicit to all team members. This may also need reinforcement from more senior managers and certainly the issue of workload may need senior management involvement to prevent the practitioner being torn in different directions.

For the researcher/practitioner

From the researcher/practitioner perspective, there are similar disadvantages to this model, relating to issues such as dissonance, boundaries and workload. Dissonance results from the conflict felt when trying to separate the roles of researcher and clinical leader or practitioner. This is obviously intertwined with the problems of workload where the practitioner '*is torn between the needs of patients and the need to be the impartial researcher*'. An inner turmoil can be created for those involved which can lead to some conflict among the team if the practitioner is not seen to be fulfilling their expectations.

One solution to this is to identify, before establishing the post, the time to be allocated to each part of the role and for all the team members to be signed up to this. Nevertheless, in times when the clinical demands are high, it is difficult to retain this perspective without being physically removed from the unit.

For clinical care

The only possible difficulty which could be seen as far as clinical care is concerned relates to the enormous workload which can be generated within the unified model, with the subsequent risk of highly pressured staff. However, with skilled management of time and resources, this can be avoided. Indeed, the chance for patients and clients to become partners in research far outweighs this potential difficulty.

Discussion

The people selected for this role need a wide array of clinical, academic and managerial skills, if the post is to be successful. They need to be competent in terms of clinical practice, leadership, change management and communication, as well as having the underpinning knowledge of the research process to undertake specific projects and help other team members to do this. As they say, '*There are times when I wonder what comes next … but having overall responsibility does give you the chance to co-ordinate more effectively. It doesn't mean you have got to do everything yourself, but you can influence the whole picture.*' This again supports the notion that this type of practitioner is developing at the leading edge of clinical practice and fits the notion of 'advanced practice' roles.

It also opens up the opportunity for seeking formal links with institutes of education as the role can provide a formal 'bridge' between research and practice. Primarily, though, the greatest advantage is that there is '*true integration and while research can inform practice so the reality of practice can inform research.*'

Resources

With increasing pressures on time and funds in both academic and clinical organisations, some difficulty can be experienced in accessing resources in a collaborative way. However, this is by no means insurmountable and contractual agreements can be explored to this end.

Transferability

This is a model which has been widely used in medicine for many years and has stood the test of time in ensuring that the clinical expertise of experienced practitioners is not lost to patients. That it can work is demonstrated by the increasing number of people working as lecturers/practitioners although as yet only a few have managerial authority for practice.[18] Hopefully, as more is learned about the way in which such roles can be managed, their number will increase.

This model has many advantages in terms of integrating research and clinical practice but should not be entered into lightly. It needs clear planning and management before being established to ensure that its full potential is met.

Model 5
External consultants

Four possible types of role have been identified under the heading of 'external consultant'.

First, the individual may be a member of the clinical team who has a part-time contract to undertake the role of consultant. The post therefore includes acting as a project leader and facilitator for specific topics. The individual then uses his/her skills to develop research assistants within the clinical area and more or less acts as an academic supervisor.

In the second type of role, the individual is employed by the unit/Trust to undertake research in various departments and is therefore external to the team involved in the study. This type of role is seen as evolutionary with continual evaluation and further development as time progresses. It is also a means to develop action research within teams who do not have the necessary research skills to do this.

The third type is the formal model of academic supervisor where the individual is employed by an academic institution but contracted to the unit/Trust for specific projects. This again requires the supervisor to develop and facilitate team members as well as offering advice on research design.

The fourth type of role refers to a situation whereby an external consultant is employed on a fixed basis by a clinical team to undertake a specific evaluation.

Strengths of the model

For the clinical team

All of these types of external consultancy have the potential to develop clinical team members' research understanding and ability to undertake evaluative projects. The presence of the consultant evaluating the team's work appears to increase the team's ability to be reflective. It also enhances cross-fertilisation with other teams/specialities, particularly when the researcher is working with more than one team at a time. For team members, *'having a researcher who we know has opened our eyes to the need to be more research-aware ourselves.'*

With the right skills it should be possible for the team members to be facilitated to act for themselves, although this may need to be negotiated as part of the agreement. In this way, they feel more involved with any research being undertaken and develop their own skills for future use within the clinical setting. This could clearly be seen as the extra value element for using this type of model.

The presence of a consultant within the team who has specialist knowledge also means that access to new information can be obtained much earlier than relying on each individual picking up information from journals and other sources. As they see it, *'We have access to a real resource of our own.'* The presence of an external consultant also encourages the clinical team to develop their ability to reflect on their practice, particularly when combined with ready access to research knowledge.

For the consultant

The consultants have easier access themselves to academic validation, supervision and support, which can be difficult to achieve for staff employed full time by a unit/Trust. This also reduces the potential for them to become an isolated researcher, which can create problems for the person as well as the quality of the research undertaken.

There is also a feeling that this model would ensure that there is methodological sympathy in the approach taken since *'through close working relationships with the clinical team you can become very "aware" of the reality of practice.'* In turn, the consultant can also help to increase the team's access to new information in order that they too have a sympathy for the constraints of research. This model also helps to ensure that the researcher is more objective than if he/she were an integral team member, as long as the risk of 'going native' is guarded against.

For practice

As with the other models, for the patients the greatest advantage is that the nurses who work with them have an increased awareness of research and the knowledge base for practice. Thus the care which patients receive is drawn from a wider range of information which should lead to greater choice.

Disadvantages of the model

For the clinical team

There may be a perception of threat from team members, particularly if they feel they are being inspected. An external consultant can also be a threat to the managers of the clinical team with whom they are working since they could be perceived as criticising the way in which they manage. Concern can arise that the consultant will come up with results which will create a conflict of interest as far as resources or service delivery are concerned. On the other hand, there is also the possibility that an external consultant may be seen as a management 'stooge' by the clinical staff, which can reduce their participation in the research process and possibly their ownership of the results.

As the external consultants agree, '*It is really important to get people on board and negotiate the way in which you will work.*' Otherwise there is some danger that any findings will not be utilised because staff do not feel part of a process which was undertaken by an outsider. This may also be a problem because the consultant is only there for a short time, which can limit the opportunity for consolidation.

For the consultant

As far as the consultant is concerned, being seen as a resource to the team in terms of facilitating their development may mean that the staff expect constant access. This can create problems not only in terms of total workload but also in being allowed to have defined time to undertake the research/evaluation. Another point relates to ethical considerations since, as one researcher pointed out, '*ethical clearance can be more problematic if the researcher is outside the Trust*'.

For practice

The only disadvantage for practice relates to the time element and the possibility of conflict arising between clinical and research priorities.

Discussion

Using this approach can lead to an increase in research awareness and research skills at a clinical level, as well as the development of sound enquiry, since the research skills are available to the team through the consultant. It also opens up the opportunity to explore systems of reciprocity between academic institutions and clinical settings, which may overcome some of the funding difficulties. As far as the researcher is concerned, there is a clear advantage '*of forging close links with practitioners and patients in order to retain a grasp of reality which can inform future practice.*' In the same way, the practitioners may get a 'taste' of research which will not only inform their current practice but may also open up career path options.

This approach also offers the opportunity for '*handling of confidential data and sensitive issues in a way which can protect confidentiality but is close enough to the team to be fed back and acted on*'. Since the researcher and team come to know each other well, mutual respect and trust can enhance the way in which they interrelate.

Threats relate to the limited time which the consultant can spend with the team, and this can constrain the impact through lack of continuity. If the work is undertaken in relative isolation from team members, the strength of the impact can be lost with the exercise seen as a peripheral activity not impacting on practice. However, this has not been found to be the case where the working relationship is sound and there is a high degree of involvement.

Resources

One difficulty with this model relates to the high cost of employing consultants even from within a university setting, which may clearly be a big problem in the current financial climate. Because the contract can be on a short-term basis, the time available can be matched to a specific work area, rather than taking on a full-time commitment.

Transferability

This is an approach which is widely used in other areas of health care, with an increase in the use of management consultants. The advantage of using consultants for practice development has not been that high to date in either nursing or other disciplines but can offer a very attractive option for either uniprofessional or multiprofessional work.

In summary, this model encompasses a number of different roles, the common theme being that an individual is brought in to undertake specific work within a clinical team. There can be advantages to this approach in relation to both funding and academic credibility, but care must be taken to ensure integration for the duration of the project.

Model 6
External researchers

This model is based upon an experienced researcher, usually based within an academic department, who is commissioned by the organisation/clinical team to undertake clearly identified research. The researcher is responsible for managing the research programme independently but is expected to collaborate closely with the clinical team. The researcher is also able to provide general research advice to the clinical team, although time for this may be limited if the actual research takes up most of their allocated time. Nevertheless *'researchers are seen at the coalface – not as dry, crusty academics in ivory towers.'* Thus it can increase access for practitioners to a 'specialist' field of nursing work which is sometimes seen as distant to others.

Strengths of the model

For the clinical team

There are clear advantages to this model in terms of access to an experienced researcher and related academic department with all its relevant resources. This increases the likelihood that the quality of the research undertaken is of a high standard. There is also an advantage to be gained in terms of credibility if a recognised researcher is carrying out the project. Frequently, clinical staff attempt to carry out research projects but their contribution can be devalued, despite its inherent quality, because they do not have academic standing. Research undertaken in this collaborative manner avoids this problem. Clearly the academic department also benefits because it has easier access to the clinical setting required for the particular research project. In turn, this can benefit the team who have greater access to the university's facilities.

For the researcher

As far as the researcher is concerned, this model has obvious benefits because the individuals *'have greater autonomy than if employed by the health organisation.'* This also provides greater flexibility in terms of planning and carrying out any project. The individuals are also less isolated from academic peers because there are still close links with the employing academic department. Thus *'collegial supervision, support and the opportunity for theory development are enhanced.'* These attributes are highly treasured by researchers and are often not possible when the researcher is employed by the health organisation funding the research. The researchers also find this generally a more fruitful pathway as far as career progression is concerned because they are constantly building their research expertise and status within an academic framework. This is not always the case for a researcher employed within the health organisation where research is not necessarily seen as a permanent career pathway.

'Access is one of the major barriers for independent researchers, so any reduction in this difficulty is welcomed.' Access not only relates to the simple issue of finding an organisation to work in but also to the co-operation of the staff working there. If the staff are not co-operative, the whole research project may and often does fail.

For practice

The greatest advantage for practice is that the end product of this approach is likely to increase the overall body of nursing knowledge, which can have long-term effects on the quality of care offered to patients. A peripheral advantage may be an increased awareness of the importance of research among the team, which will influence future practice.

Disadvantages of the model

For the clinical team

With regard to the clinical staff, there is always the danger with this model that they feel excluded from the research being undertaken. There can be a feeling of elitism that they could not possibly understand what the researcher is doing, which then creates fear and mistrust. All these problems can reduce their desire to co-operate, and this will affect the quality of the research. The clinical staff may also refuse to implement any changes suggested by the research because they do not feel any ownership of the process.

For the researcher

As far as the researcher is concerned, there is *'the never-ending problem of gaining support from clinical and managerial staff'*. Sometimes a researcher is employed by one senior individual without the full co-operation of all the other members of staff. This creates difficulties for the researcher who has to persuade the team to participate and see the value of the particular project. There is also the difficulty of competing demands as far as the clinical staff are concerned. The researcher may request their time and find that patient needs override this. As they say, *'This is not only cost-ineffective, it is also very frustrating for a researcher.'*

For patient care

As the outcomes of work of this nature may take some time to be evident, it is less likely that the patients or clients who participate in the research will be the major benefactors, although most people are more than happy to participate in work which will help others in the future. There is also a need to give consideration to ethical clearance and ensure that any involvement is informed fully.

Discussion

This model gives the unit access to a high level of expertise and rigour in the manner in which the research is conducted. It also provides access to the research support systems available within a university, such as statistical analysis and library search facilities. Furthermore, through their position within academic departments, the researches have a ready way of *'getting into the research circuit, are established in public speaking and often known to conference organisers'*.

There are, however, times when the pace of the research and the pace of the development work do not coincide, which may result in one or other being delayed. For example, the researcher may require time to gather baseline data before changes are made in practice, while the clinicians may be ready to move forward, and feel a sense of frustration at being held back. Ways of overcoming such difficulties include constant feedback, interim reports and use of focus groups.

There is also the risk of distancing between the researcher and practitioner, and great care has to be taken to retain effective communication between the two parties. This is balanced to some extent by the advantage of having a more objective external perspective.

Other difficulties with this model relate to issues such as cost and co-operation.

Resources

External researchers are costly, particularly when one considers the overhead charges from the host university. Balanced against this, however, must be the time-limited nature of this commitment; one only pays for the particular piece of work, not a permanent member of staff. It can be difficult to persuade senior managers that employing an external researcher provides value for money, particularly if they do not fully understand the need for high-quality research.

Transferability

This is a well-tested model of research which has been used in other fields for many years. With an increase in emphasis on multi-professional work, it opens up the opportunity for collaboration between disciplines, working from a shared base. However, it is important to recognise the contribution which each individual profession brings to a particular issue, although this must be done within a multiprofessional context.

This model works well in terms of developing strong academic links, ensuring career development for the researcher and access to academic resources for the practitioners. With good collaboration, it provides the opportunity for sound research as well as ownership by the clinical team.

Discussion

The models described above are not mutually exclusive but offer a range of ways in which research and practice can be brought together. There does not appear to be a perfect approach as all have both advantages and disadvantages. However, an awareness of the potential pitfalls means that strategies can be developed to minimise them.

Similarly, none of the reasons for gathering information and undertaking enquiry in clinical practice is exclusive but each does require a differing approach. Clarity about the type of information which is both needed and expected can go some way towards identifying the structures, skills and organisational expectations which arise from the differing requirements.

If effective ways are to be found to bring together research and practice in order that patients or clients receive the most appropriate care, based on sound knowledge, then an investment must be made in providing organisational opportunities and resources for this to occur. From widespread evidence of the lack of use of research in practice (in nursing and other disciplines), it can be argued that circulation of empirical knowledge through literature is not an effective precursor of change alone, although it does have an important role to play. Neither have tightly formulated, centrally developed protocols or procedures been widely influential in practice and in some instances may have created a gap between espoused and used theory.

If we are to truly influence the manner in which service is developed, there is a need to find creative ways of providing the opportunity for development which recognise the imperatives of both service provision and scientific enquiry. Of the models described above, the opportunities to develop unified roles, to have access to research skills within the team, or to develop partnerships between academic and clinical sites seem to be the most exciting, since they bring together the expertise from both settings and can meet both the developmental and research needs most fully. Not only does this address the issue of interface and ensure that there is a mutual respect, but it also offers an excellent opportunity in relation to the development of a clinical career path. In this way, competences can be identified apart from an extension of managerial responsibility which could be used to develop roles and allow our expert practitioners to stay in practice while advancing their careers.

The skills required to fulfil these roles should not, however, be underestimated, since the demand of such work is complex. Furthermore, it is essential that work of this nature is undertaken with rigour in order to gain credibility among a wide audience.

This does not underestimate the value of internal roles which are very often a much more appropriate starting point to initiate research awareness and use in practice. In some ways, this work is even more challenging as there may well be some resistance to the changes which are required in practice.

While 'empowerment' may be an overused word at the moment, there is no doubt that the involvement of staff in development, where an ethos is created which encourages exploration, is one of the most critical factors in taking practice forward. Investing in strong clinical leadership, differentiated from the equally important need for managerial leadership, is one way of ensuring that such empowerment can occur. Within all these models this has been a central feature without which the success of the work may have been less evident.

A future model which may be explored is for a clinical unit to act as a central source of expertise for other nurses within the Trust, taking the lead in providing advice and direction to the Trust's overall research and development (R&D) strategy in relation to nursing issues. Both the unified-roles model and the researcher internal to the team offer great potential here. Thus the development of a clinical research unit with strong formal academic links could evolve to undertake rigorous practice-driven research. There is no doubt that this would theoretically provide an excellent way of ensuring that the research and development strategy of the organisation was practice-driven and hence grounded in reality. Much would also be gained from such work being undertaken within a multiprofessional context where the contribution of nursing can be explored in relation to the rest of the clinical team. Indeed, this is one way in which the knowledge and experience of practitioners can help to contribute to strategic planning. It is, however, a vast role and consideration would have to be given to resource implications and the background of the incumbents. Care must also be taken to avoid units of this nature becoming isolated from the rest of an organisation and hence being perceived as elitist or unrealistic.

The challenges which are faced in moving towards a more effective practice-research interface are numerous and require a balance between managerial and scientific imperatives. The models described here can be seen as a continuum of development relating to the needs of the organisation, the current stage of development and the confidence and competence of those involved. The experiences gained through overviewing a number of different approaches and considering the implications could act as a useful discussion point in taking forward the proposals within both local and national R&D strategies.

While there has been a strong emphasis on the co-ordination and dissemination of knowledge related to clinical effectiveness, less attention has been paid to ways in which local, context-driven initiatives can translate this information into clinical action. Hopefully, the points raised in this publication will contribute to widespread debate around this area. Discussion of the viability of the different options and the sharing of experiences of the effectiveness of differing approaches would be of widespread value to both the professions and, more importantly, to service delivery.

References

1. Department of Health. Report of the Taskforce on the Strategy for Research in Nursing, Midwifery and Health Visiting. London: DoH, 1993.

2. Department of Health. Improving the effectiveness of the NHS. Executive Letter 74. London: DoH, 1994.

3. See 2.

4. Department of Health. The Evolution of Clinical Audit. London: DoH, 1994.

5.Department of Health. A Vision for the Future. London: DoH, 1993.

6. Turner Shaw J, Bosanquet N. A Way to Develop Nurses and Nursing. London: King's Fund Centre, 1993.

7. See 1.

8. United Kingdom Central Council for Nursing, Midwifery and Health Visiting. The Report of the Post-Registration Education and Practice Project. London: UKCC, 1990.

9. Knowles M. The Adult Learner: A neglected species. Houston: Gulf, 1990.

10.See 4.

11. See 8.

12. Wandelt M, Ager J. Quality Patient Care Scale. New York: Appleton-Century-Crofts, 1974.

13. Herbert R, Evans A. Staff Appraisal and Development. Senior Nurse 1991; 11(6):9-11

14. Kohner N. Clinical Supervision in Practice. London: King's Fund, 1994.

15. See 8.

16. Sheppard B. Looking Back – Moving Forward: Developing elderly care rehabilitation and the nurse's role within it. Brighton: Brighton Health Care NHS Trust, 1994.

17. Pearson A. The Clinical Nursing Unit. London: William Heinemann Medical Books Ltd, 1983.

18. Lathlean J, Vaughan B. Unifying Nursing Practice and Theory. Oxford: Butterworth-Heinemann Ltd Health Service, 1994.

Appendix
Workshop participants

Anne Appadoo	Ward Manager, Truth Ward NDU, North Middlesex Hospital
Gillian Bell	Ward Sister, Ward 33/CCU, Glenfield Hospital
Val Buxton	Health Visitor, Stepney NDU, Steels Lane Health Centre
Clare Byrne	Clinical Research Facilitator, Liverpool NDU, Royal Liverpool University Hospital
Usha Chandran	Practice Development Nurse, Annex NDU, St George's Hospital
Jimmy Cooper	Clinical Leader, Brighton Critical Care NDU, Royal Sussex County Hospital
Margaret Dennerly	Staff Nurse/RGN, Liverpool NDU, Royal Liverpool University Hospital
Clare Dikken	Clinical Leader, Day Ward NDU, Worthing Hospital
Tom Dodd	Acute CPN Office, Michael Flanagan NDU
Amanda Evans	NDU Leader, Byron Ward NDU, King's Healthcare
Angus Forbes	Health Visitor/District Nurse, Stepney NDU, Steels Lane Health Centre
Sarah Furlong	Researcher, Ward 33/CCU, Glenfield Hospital
Rob Garbett	Project Worker, Ward 7e NDU, John Radcliffe Hospital

Peter Griffiths	Researcher, Byron Ward NDU, KIng's Healthcare
Claire Hale	Centre for Health Services Research, University of Newcastle-upon-Tyne
Christine Halek	Clinical Leader, Annex NDU, St George's Hospital
Ruth Harris	Sister, Byron Ward NDU, King's Healthcare
Brenda Hawkey	Clinical Leader, Homeward Rehabilitation NDU, Brigton General Hospital
Sam Keyes	Senior Staff Nurse, ITU, Chelsea & Westminster Hospital
Sylvain Laxade	Clinical Leader, Royal Victoria Infirmary NDU, Newcastle
Kim Manley	Clinical Nursing Specialist, ITU, Chelsea & Westminster Hospital
Carolyn Mills	Clinical Leader, Truth Ward NDU, North Middlesex Hospital
Lisa Otter	Liverpool NDU, Royal Liverpool University Hospital
Julie Scholes	Project Leader – Researcher, Brighton Critical Care NDU, Royal Sussex County Hospital
Barbara Sheppard	Researcher, Day Ward NDU, Worthing Hospital
John Sitzia	Researcher, Day Ward NDU, Worthing Hospital
Susan Waterworth	Clinical Leader, Liverpool NDU, Royal Liverpool University Hospital